SIRTFOOD DIET FOR WOMEN

PLAN YOUR WEIGHT LOSS WITH SIRTUIN ACTIVATOR RECIPES

HALEY JOSEPH

CONTENTS

Introduction v

1. Benefits of the Sirtfood Diet 1
2. Sirtfood Diet and Exercise 9
3. The Sirtfood Lifestyle 17
4. Breakfast Recipes 21
5. Lunch Recipes 33
6. Dinner Recipes 45
7. Snack Recipes 61
8. Dessert Recipes 71

Afterword 81

© Copyright 2020 by:- Haley Joseph All rights reserved.

The content contained within this book may not be reproduced, duplicated or transmitted without direct written permission from the author or the publisher.

Under no circumstances will any blame or legal responsibility be held against the publisher, or author, for any damages, reparation, or monetary loss due to the information contained within this book, either directly or indirectly.

Legal Notice:

This book is copyright protected. It is only for personal use. You cannot amend, distribute, sell, use, quote or paraphrase any part, or the content within this book, without the consent of the author or publisher.

Disclaimer Notice:

Please note the information contained within this document is for educational and entertainment purposes only. All effort has been executed to present accurate, up to date, reliable, complete information. No warranties of any kind are declared or implied. Readers acknowledge that the author is not engaging in the rendering of legal, financial, medical or professional advice. The content within this book has been derived from various sources. Please consult a licensed professional before attempting any techniques outlined in this book.

By reading this document, the reader agrees that under no circumstances is the author responsible for any losses, direct or indirect, that are incurred as a result of the use of information contained within this document, including, but not limited to, errors, omissions, or inaccuracies.

INTRODUCTION

Have you been struggling to lose weight?

Have you tried several different diets but with no success?

Are you looking for a solution to your weight loss issues?

Well, if the answer is yes, this is the right book for you!

The modern-day diet and overall lifestyle have negatively impacted most people's health. Everyone leads a busy life with too much work and too many responsibilities, with seemingly too little time to do much else. People eat out at restaurants or order take-out and junk food a lot more frequently than they ever cook a healthy meal at home. With the unhealthy lifestyle most of us have been living, gaining extra weight seems to be inevitable. However, people have become a lot more conscious of the negative impact of this unhealthy lifestyle in recent times.

No one really wants to gain those extra pounds and deal with the other side effects of weight gain. However, it can be really difficult to lose weight and get back on track. This is

Introduction

especially true if you are following all the wrong diets that are out there. Most of the fad diets tell people to eat too little, skip meals, use a nutrient-deficit meal plan, or exercise too much. While you may have tried these for a while, you will notice that they do more harm than good. If you eat too little, you will eventually give in to hunger and end up binge eating. If you stick to a select number of foods, you will get bored and you won't take in all the nutrients your body requires either. If you go on a liquid cleanse, it will mess up your digestive system.

All such diets might give you temporary weight loss results, but you will pile on the pounds as soon as you stop following them again. They also require you to exert a lot of self-control and discipline, which can be difficult. If you have tried all of this and agree with us, then we'll tell you exactly what you need to change and how to achieve the results you are looking for.

This is where the Sirtfood diet comes in. The diet is named after the sirtuin activators present in certain foods. These molecules help to protect cells from inflammation, aging, and other unwanted metabolic processes. This is why sirtuin activators are linked to longevity and other benefits that you will learn about in this book. More importantly for you, they help with weight loss. Unlike other fad diets, the Sirtfood diet does not focus on helping you lose weight solely by trying some tricks. Instead, the diet will help you eat better for the long term so you can lose extra weight and maintain a healthy body without compromising. Sirtuin activators are present in a lot of different foods so you will be able to enjoy a diverse diet.

Introduction

Along with changes in diet, you will also learn how to improve your eating habits and overall lifestyle to facilitate the weight loss process. Anyone can follow the Sirtfood diet since it is not very restrictive, expensive, or difficult to follow. If you have any underlying health conditions, you can always consult your doctor first to see if the diet is currently suitable for you. If not, this diet will not have any negative effects on your health.

This book will help you learn all that you need to know about the Sirtfood diet. It will help you understand what Sirtfoods are and how they help you. You will learn about the various benefits of the diet. It will also tell you about how you can implement the diet with other positive lifestyle changes in a simple but effective way. More importantly, this book has several Sirtfood recipes to help you get started. It will ensure that you prepare delicious but healthy meals that benefit your body. The information on Sirt foods in this book will be more than enough to help you begin your switch from the unhealthy lifestyle that made you gain extra weight to a healthy one with your body in the best shape it has ever been.

Studies show that a majority of the population finds it difficult to figure out how they can eat healthy while losing weight. This is why it is important to adopt a diet that is not like other fad eating plans. These are completely useless and sometimes even harmful. Each person has a different body type and something that works for one person might not work for another.

Some people find it a lot easier to lose weight compared to others whose bodies stubbornly retain weight—even if they do the same things. However, the Sirtfood diet can help

Introduction

surpass such issues in a better way. Even if you have struggled with weight loss for a long time, the guidelines of this diet will help you achieve results. Once you combine a Sirtfood diet with a healthy exercise regimen, there is nothing that will prevent you from getting back into shape. But you may still be wondering: how does this diet work and what will it do for me?

The Sirtfood diet was originally launched in 2016 by Aiden Goggins and Glen Matten. These two nutritionists from the United Kingdom wrote a book on a diet that they claimed would activate the skinny gene in anyone so they could burn fat a lot faster. It soon became extremely popular and celebrities like Adele and Pippa Middleton began to follow it. The term Sirt itself is an abbreviated form of sirtuins, which you will learn more about later. The Sirtfood diet plan claims to help people with weight loss, higher energy levels, and better health in the long run.

The diet is primarily based on consuming foods that are rich in sirtuin activators. Sirtuins are proteins in the body that play a very important role. There are seven different sirtuins in all mammals: Sirt-1, Sirt-2, Sirt-3, Sirt-4, Sirt-5, Sirt-6, and Sirt-7. They help to protect your cells, reduce signs of aging, increase energy efficiency, and also make you more resistant to stress.

To benefit from these sirtuins, you have to consume foods that will activate their function. These two nutritionists conducted a lot of research over the years until they figured out a list of Sirtfoods and a plan that would help people benefit from them. According to studies on the people found to have the greatest longevity in the world, it was

Introduction

evident that a plant-rich diet is an important factor to healthy eating.

People in these regions—the blue zones—consumed nearly five times the amount of plant-based foods as people in other places. The polyphenol content in this kind of diet is a major factor, but the founders of the Sirtfood diet found that certain types of polyphenols were more effective than others. That small group of polyphenols activated the sirtuins or skinny genes in the body to mimic the benefits of exercise and fasting. This is why it is important to have foods that have more sirtuin-activating polyphenols. Sirtuins have seven proteins and they are activated when you consume certain plant compounds and foods. These will trigger chemical pathways in your body that will further promote weight loss.

You can see the evidence of the benefits of Sirtfoods if you look at the blue zones around the world. These are the regions that have demonstrated the highest longevity compared to other places around the world. The people living in blue zones live a much longer and healthier life. The highest number of centenarians can be found in these blue zones. Not only do they live longer, but they also have higher levels of energy and retain vigor throughout their lives. However, people in other places who follow the modern-day lifestyle tend to age much faster and become ill in their advanced years.

While people in other places suffer from diseases, lose energy, and have a lower quality of life over the years, it is the opposite for those in blue zones. These people show fewer signs of a decrease in cognitive abilities. Even people above 100 can be seen walking around instead of being

Introduction

bedridden. Most of the blue zones are around the Mediterranean Sea, in Japan, Costa Rica, and Italy.

The blue zones have something in common: their diet. The diets of these blue zones have a high number of Sirtfoods. While people assume that the Mediterranean diet is all about pasta or pizza, people in these regions actually consume very little of such foods. Sirtfoods like fish and olive oil are more prominent in their daily diet. People in Japan also prefer seafood and consume a lot of green tea, which is high in antioxidants. In Costa Rica, dark cocoa and coffee are common foods. The point is that the people in these blue zones are a prime example of the benefits of the Sirtfood diet. This diet is not just some strict food or exercise plan. For them, it is a way of life and how they eat regularly. This is why they can reap all the benefits of this healthy diet in the long run.

The diet helps to identify a group of foods that works to activate the sirtuins in your body. Having a diet specifically rich in these foods showed stunning results in the people who first tried it out. On average, they lost about 7 pounds in a week. This helped the nutritionists realize that the diet really works. The skinny gene or Sirt 1 is a sirtuin that helps to regulate metabolic activities and the storage of fat. They were then able to figure out a Sirtfood diet plan from which everyone could benefit.

The Sirtfood diet is not meant to help people solely with weight loss; it has other benefits as well. Even though there isn't a lot of scientific evidence to back all the claims of the Sirtfood diet, people who have tried it generally vouch for its effectiveness. It helps to regulate both metabolic and physiological functions in the body that will increase

Introduction

longevity, reduce inflammation, and improve digestion. Certain studies have also shown that the Sirt gene helps to protect the cardiovascular system in the body because of its anti-inflammatory effect. While a lot more research still has to be conducted to confirm such claims, they seem to run in favor of the Sirtfood diet.

CHAPTER 1

BENEFITS OF THE SIRTFOOD DIET

According to various studies, the Sirtfood diet is quite beneficial for your health. Here are just some of those benefits:

- The sirtuin activators work in a way that allows you to suppress an unhealthy appetite, lose extra weight, and build more muscle. This is one of the primary reasons why women all over the world have been trying this diet. It allows weight loss without having to starve or skip meals. This diet also helps adherents to lose weight while retaining or building muscle loss if the right exercise routine is followed. It will allow you to look toned while losing weight instead of looking too skinny or sallow. While other fad diets may result in a lot of muscle loss, this diet actually promotes the growth of more muscle.
- The diet also has a positive effect on your focus, concentration, and memory.
- Sirtfoods can help in blood sugar regulation. It is

beneficial for people who suffer or are at risk for diseases like diabetes type 2. The modern diet, on the other hand, makes people more prone to blood sugar issues.

- The Sirtfood diet protects the body against damage from free radicals. These free radicals cause faster aging and also make the body more prone to diseases like cancer. Studies have shown that consuming more foods rich in sirtuin activators can help to reduce the risk of such chronic diseases. Frank Hu, a professor from Harvard University, also endorsed this particular benefit of the diet.
- The diet is a lot more flexible compared to other diets. You don't have to spend a lot of money on expensive ingredients either. You just need to consume more wholesome foods that are high in sirtuin activators. This includes foods like bananas, tomatoes, turmeric, kale, etc. which are all easy-to-find ingredients.
- Sirtfoods will benefit your health even if you don't follow the diet down to every detail. Just by incorporating more Sirtfoods into your diet, you will increase your ability to burn fat and reap the other benefits of these sirtuin activators.

Top 10 Sirtfoods

Dark chocolate

Dark chocolate that has at least 70% of unprocessed cocoa is a great Sirtfood. It is a rich source of flavonoids and is beneficial for health in many ways. If you have a sweet tooth, you can have a bite of dark chocolate to curb cravings while following the diet. It also helps to boost serotonin and endorphin levels in the body. Dark chocolate has chemicals that are said to reduce the risk of heart disease, stroke, and even high blood pressure.

Red wine

A glass of red wine a day is beneficial for your health, though more than this will do more harm than good. Red wine has antioxidants and is also anti-inflammatory. It is made from grape seeds and skins and has a high amount of polyphenols. It also contains resveratrol, which is good for women. These contents in red wine help to reduce levels of bad cholesterol, prevent the formation of blood clots, and protect the blood vessels. As long as it is consumed in moderation, red wine is considered a superfood.

Onions

Onions have a high content of antioxidants and thus boost the immune system. Onions also have a lot of vitamin C. They are very low in calories but add a lot of flavor to any meal. They contain quercetin, which is a compound that can help protect your body against certain types of cancers.

Green tea

Green tea is one of the few Sirtfood-friendly beverages. It is a superfood with a high amount of antioxidants. It helps to protect the cells in the body from damage. The catechins in green tea improve metabolic rates and promote weight loss. Matcha green tea is the most beneficial form that you can consume and is very popular in Japan.

Blueberries

Blueberries are another food with a high antioxidant count. It has various benefits like reducing inflammation, reducing signs of aging, lowering levels of bad cholesterol, and also burning fat. This Sirtfood is rich in phytonutrients and can be enjoyed as a daily snack.

Coffee

You don't have to cut off coffee on the Sirtfood diet, as long as you don't add additives like sugar. A cup of coffee will make you energetic and increases endurance. It also has the potential to improve brain function and protect against certain diseases.

Parsley

Parsley has a high amount of chlorophyll, which has great antioxidant properties. It also contains alpha-linolenic acid, which reduces the risk of heart disease. Parsley is a great ingredient for those who have arthritis or are showing early signs of it. It contains luteolin, which is good for maintaining eye health.

Turmeric

Turmeric is a superfood that has various beneficial properties. It works as an antiseptic and is also anti-inflammatory. This spice is rich in antioxidants. Turmeric contains a compound called curcumin, which gives it the yellow color and also helps to prevent cancer, Alzheimer's, and blood clots.

Olive oil

Olive oil is a Sirtfood diet-friendly ingredient that is better than other refined oils. It helps to lower levels of bad cholesterol in the body. It also contains a lot of monounsaturated fatty acids and this helps to regulate blood sugar and insulin. It can be added to salads or used for stir-frying foods without adding too many calories to your daily intake.

Other Sirtfood diet-friendly ingredients are:

- Greens like kale, asparagus, bok choy, broccoli, watercress, spinach, celery, parsley
- Fruits like blackberries, black plums, red grapes, cranberries, raspberries, strawberries, mulberries, apple, kiwi, Medjool dates, lemons, pomegranate
- Vegetables like shallots, white onions, capers, olives, artichokes, arugula, garlic, red onions, seaweed, spirulina, horseradish, crimini mushrooms, cabbage, cucumber, edamame, tomato, ginger, peppers, natto beans, beets
- Spices like chili, capers, cloves, cumin, cinnamon
- Nuts and seeds like almonds, chestnuts, pecans, pistachios, sunflower seeds, walnuts
- Herbs like dill, oregano, sage, chives, peppermint, thyme, basil, rosemary
- Beverages like black coffee, green tea, water, fresh green juices
- Other miscellaneous foods like soy, buckwheat, quinoa, olive oil

Sirtfood Diet Plan

Using the Sirtfood list given above, you can create a meal plan for yourself as you follow the Sirtfood diet.

. . .

Phase 1

This is the hyper success phase. It will last for seven days. For three days, you have to limit yourself to 1000 calories. You can have three green juices with one Sirtfood rich meal on these days. For the next four days, you are allowed to consume 1500 calories. On these days, you can enjoy two Sirtfood rich meals and two green juices.

Phase 2

This is the maintenance phase. It will last for 14 days and it is during this phase that you will steadily lose weight. On these days, you will be consuming one green juice and three Sirtfood rich meals.

Post Both Phases

Once you have completed the first two phases of the Sirtfood diet, you can be less strict about following the diet. The initial two phases of the Sirtfood diet help kick start its effects on your body. After these three weeks, you are encouraged to continue consuming a Sirtfood-rich diet along with a glass of green juice every day. You can use the list of Sirt foods to help guide you along, plus the recipes in the book for inspiration. You will start observing sustainable weight loss during the initial weeks, but if you continue eating a diet rich in Sirtfoods, the weight loss will continue. The diet is not a one-off plan that you need to stop after three weeks—only to revert to your old eating habits. Stopping abruptly will make it easy to put all the weight back on and will also prevent you from reaping the other benefits of the diet. However, by incorporating a simpler version of the diet with more Sirtfoods into your regular eating habits, you can see long-term benefits.

This is an example of a day on the Sirtfood diet:

- Breakfast: Soy yogurt topped with chopped walnuts and mixed berries.
- Lunch: Salad made with kale, celery, parsley, and apple. Top it off with walnuts. Drizzle some lemon juice and olive oil over the salad.
- Midday: Green Sirtfood juice made with celery, kale, green apple, ginger, matcha, etc.
- Dinner: Buckwheat noodles made with kale and stir-fried prawns.

CHAPTER 2

SIRTFOOD DIET AND EXERCISE

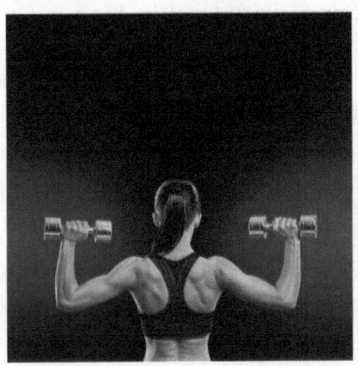

If you want to see real results, solely changing your diet is not enough. You need to start exercising regularly to help your body burn fat, build muscle, and to remain healthy for a longer time. Sitting at your desk for long hours or following any kind of sedentary lifestyle will only harm you.

The human body needs adequate exercise to remain optimally functional and in good shape. If you eat a lot of food, but your activity levels are low, the body has no way of burning energy. Instead, your food gets stored as fats and thus adds to your body weight. This is why a sedentary lifestyle makes you overweight. However, if you are active throughout the day, the body will burn more energy and thus help you lose weight. If you exercise while following the Sirtfood diets, you can increase the fat-burning process already initiated by the sirtuins.

However, it is better to reduce or stop exercising during the first phase of the Sirtfood diet. This is because the low-calorie intake may not be sufficient to give you enough energy for a high level of activity. Exercising will increase your risk of experiencing lightheadedness and fatigue. You can increase your activity level in the third week and exercise normally after the first two phases of the diet.

Exercise should become a part of your daily routine if you want to live a healthy life. It is not necessary to exercise every day of the week, but five days are recommended. You need not follow an extremely tough workout regime either. Various forms of exercise will allow you to burn off the extra weight. Swimming, running, cycling, and playing sports like basketball or tennis are a great way to burn a lot of calories in a short time. You can also alternate with lighter exercise like a walk or some yoga, which is slow-paced but very effective.

If you really want to push your body into the fat-burning mode, there are great workout routines that you can follow online or sign up for at a gym. As long as you keep your body moving, you will be able to burn calories. Even if you skip a few days of exercise, don't allow yourself to be demotivated. You can always get right back on track. The Sirtfoods will help you see results quite quickly and this itself will act as motivation to help you follow a healthier lifestyle.

While exercising, you need to ensure that you add protein to your diet. Have some protein about an hour after you finish your workout. While exercise can make your muscles sore and strained, the protein will help to repair them and aid in recovery. Recipes with a high amount of protein are perfect for an after-workout snack or meal. For instance, you can make the Sirt chili con carne or a salad with chicken and greens. If you prefer a smoothie after working out, mix greens with blueberries and add a scoop of protein powder. It is up to you to decide on the kind of workout you prefer.

The Sirtfood diet will help you change your eating habits, burn fat, and improve overall health. You might find the diet challenging in the initial phase, but it gets a lot easier after that. The only detail you need to pay attention to is including Sirtfoods in your diet. Your body will take a little time to adapt so you need to be kind to yourself. Don't exercise too much and strain yourself during this period. You can slowly implement a workout routine and increase the intensity level after the first two weeks. This change in diet along with regular exercise will help you lose weight, increase your energy levels throughout the day, and sleep better at night. The effectiveness of the diet differs from each individual and also depends on how far you push yourself to see results.

Bodyweight Exercises

If you prefer working out at home without equipment or going to the gym, bodyweight exercises are very effective. These have been tried and tested by a lot of fitness experts and help you burn fat while building muscle. Unlike actual weights, these will not cause your body to bulk up in an unwanted way. Instead, you will watch as your body slowly gets toned and back into shape.

Bodyweight training has many benefits:

- It will speed up weight loss
- It slows down the process of aging
- It will help you improve your performance in any sport
- It will increase your self-confidence
- It helps to reduce mood swings
- It will reduce the risk of diseases
- It can be done anywhere and at any time
- It helps to improve mobility, strength, and stability

Before you begin bodyweight training, it is a good idea to plan out the workout. First, you have to decide on the frequency of your training sessions. Note down the number of sets or repetitions you want to do of a particular exercise. The intensity of the workout will also vary.

A high-intensity interval training session will be extremely intense but for about 20 minutes. A low-intensity workout should be longer in duration to make up for the lower activity level. In general, you should try to work out about 3-5 times a week. This means you will be working out for 3-5 hours a week. At least two of these workouts should focus on strength training. You also need to do some moderately intensive cardio during each session. If you want to use the Sirtfood diet and bodyweight training to maximize weight loss, you should put in more effort to burn more calories.

Although high-intensity interval training is great for losing weight, it should not be done every day. Alternate these sessions with lower-intensity forms of exercise. You need to adjust your diet to ensure that you are only consuming as many calories as you really need. Weight loss requires calorie deficit but in a healthy way. If you have a balanced diet with a good workout regimen and adequate sleep, your health will improve in no time.

The following are bodyweight exercises that will target specific regions of your body:

Total body

- Jumping jacks
- High knees
- Mountain climbers
- 4 count burpees
- Flat out burpees
- Star jacks
- Tuck jumps

Abs

- High plank
- High side plank
- Low plank
- Low side plank
- Sit-ups
- Crunches
- Bicycle crunches

- Quadruped limb raises
- Leg raises
- Scissor kicks
- Windshield wipers

Back

- Superman
- Superman pulls
- Bridge
- Quadruped limb raises
- Low plank
- Single leg bridge
- Prone X
- Single leg deadlift
- Wall lateral pull-downs

Chest

- Push-ups
- Knee push-ups
- Wide push-ups
- Alligator push-ups
- Commander push-ups
- Plyo push-ups
- Single leg push-ups

Glutes

- Hip abduction
- Bent leg cross overs
- Bridge
- Single leg bridge

- Curtsy lunge
- Donkey kicks
- Pistol squats
- Side lunges
- Plie squats
- Fire hydrant

Arms and shoulders

- Tricep dips
- Pike push-ups
- Single leg pike push-ups
- Narrow knee push-ups
- Narrow push-ups
- Declined wall push-ups

Calves

- Calf raises
- Inward calf raises
- Outward calf raises

Legs / Thighs

- Squats
- Jump squats
- Narrow squats
- Pistol squats
- 180 jump squats
- Side lunges
- Backward lunges
- Jump lunges
- SL squats

- Wall sit
- Forward lunges
- Curtsy lunges
- Single leg deadlift

You can look up any of these exercises online for instructions or even videos to guide you. Just make sure to follow the guidelines so you practice them the right way and don't injure yourself. Also, remember to warm up before your workout and wind down once you are done. If you don't do this, you will quickly end up tired and may also injure yourself. Remember not to exert yourself too much when you first begin. You can increase the intensity and duration of your workouts over time. Remember to focus on the entire body; don't do exercises for a specific part of the body for too long. A whole-body focus will help you tone up your entire body and lose weight proportionately. With the increase in Sirtfoods and bodyweight training, your body will be at its ideal weight and health very soon.

CHAPTER 3
THE SIRTFOOD LIFESTYLE

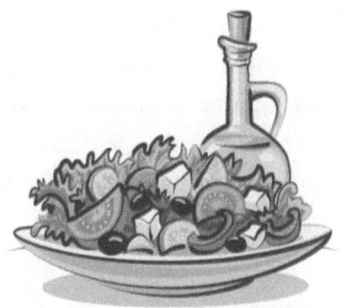

As you might have understood by now, the Sirtfood diet is more of a lifestyle. You need to adjust your diet and also exercise regularly to see it work. However, there are other small changes that you will have to keep in mind. If you can implement all the tips given here, you will be following the Sirtfood lifestyle successfully.

Mindset

Don't wait for the perfect time to begin the diet. Once you have read this book, you know enough to help you get started. The sooner you start, the faster you will see results. The perfect time never comes if you keep waiting. You need to be determined to see yourself through the entire three weeks of the diet. Once you have successfully done this, remember to follow the basic guidelines even after the three weeks. Your mindset will play an important role in this. Only you can push yourself to see it through.

Sleep Properly

A healthy sleeping schedule is crucial for a healthy body and a healthy lifestyle. You need to fix a time to go to bed and wake up every day. Don't use the excuse of having too much work to stay up late at night. You can get it done by waking up early. People with a bad sleeping schedule tend to have bad eating habits, unhealthy cravings, and gain weight faster. If you sleep better, it makes you more energetic throughout the day and will also help you make better choices for your health.

Control Your Portions

This diet does not dictate your portion size, but you need to eat the right way. If you eat too much, it will only harm your body. Use a smaller plate instead of a bigger one. This way you will feel full just by seeing the small plate piled with food instead of a big one piled with more food. Eating slowly will also help you become more conscious of the signal your brain sends you when you are full. If you eat too fast, you will end up eating much more than you really need to satisfy your hunger. Controlling portions will also help you have more control over your calorie consumption.

Support System

If you find it difficult to follow through with a diet, get someone to do it with you, or to keep you motivated. Having a support system will be encouraging and increase the likelihood of you following the diet.

These tips may be simple but are something that a lot of people fail to follow in their daily life. Being more mindful of your lifestyle will help you improve your quality of life.

Precautions

Like any new diet, you need to exercise a little precaution when you begin the Sirtfood diet. The first phase of the diet will greatly reduce the number of calories that you consume in a day and this is a cause of concern for some people. You might wonder if your body will be getting adequate nutrition and energy if you eat that way. However, this reduced calorie intake is only for a couple of days and thus doesn't have any serious impact on your health. It is only a cause of concern if you already have certain underlying health conditions that require you to eat in a specific way that does not corroborate with the Sirtfood diet.

For instance, the diet causes changes in levels of blood sugar in a way that might be harmful to patients with diabetes type 2. This is why it is important to check with a medical professional first to ensure that you can follow the diet. They may even help you adjust the diet in a way better suited for your body personally. If you don't have such health issues, the only thing you have to fight in the first phase are hunger and cravings. People who tend to eat a lot of food or consume too much sugar will find it a little tough to make the sudden switch. However, this calorie restriction is easy to overcome since it only lasts for a few days.

Another reason you might be left hungry is that you will mostly be on juices and these lack the fiber that helps to keep you full. The other side effects of this diet are short-lived and not a cause for concern. You might experience a little lightheadedness, irritability, or fatigue because of the calorie restriction. Since the diet is only for three weeks, you will not experience any serious impact on your health even if you have these side effects. However, a lot of people overcome such side effects and can make the transition to the Sirtfood diet without much effort. The only thing that you need to be prepared for initially is to fight cravings or hunger.

CHAPTER 4
BREAKFAST RECIPES

Cauliflower Kale Frittata with Green Juice

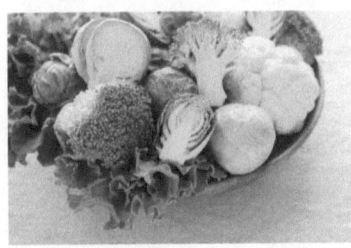

Preparation time: 10 minutes
Cooking time: 25 minutes
Number of servings: 4
Nutritional values per serving: ¼ portion with a glass juice

Frittata | Green Juice
Calories – 153.1 | Calories – 101
Fat – 5.9 g | Fat – 1 g
Carbohydrate – 6.1 g | Carbohydrate – 21 g
Protein – 19.6 g | Protein – 5 g

Ingredients:
<u>For frittata:</u>

- 2 cups chopped cauliflower
- 4 large eggs
- 12 large egg whites
- 2 tablespoons milk
- 2 cups shredded kale, discard hard ribs and stems before shredding
- ½ teaspoon garlic powder
- 3 teaspoons grated parmesan cheese
- ½ cup water
- Pepper to taste
- 1 teaspoon dried thyme
- Salt to taste

<u>For green juice:</u>

- 10.6 ounces kale leaves
- A handful parsley
- 2 green apples, cored, sliced
- Juice of 2 lemons
- 4.5 ounces rocket lettuce
- 8 celery sticks, chopped
- 2 inches ginger, sliced
- 2 teaspoons matcha green tea powder

Directions:

1. Gather all the ingredients for green juice and set it aside.
2. To make the frittata: Place a cast-iron skillet or an ovenproof skillet over medium-high flame.

3. Place cauliflower in the pan. Pour water and cook until tender.
4. Meanwhile, whisk together eggs, whites, salt, pepper, and milk in a bowl. You can use an electric hand mixer for whisking. Whisk the mixture until nice and frothy, at least 2 – 3 minutes.
5. Add garlic powder, kale, and thyme into the skillet and give it a good stir. Once the kale wilts, remove the vegetables from the pan and place it in the bowl with the egg mixture. Stir well.
6. Spray the skillet with cooking spray and pour the egg mixture into the skillet. Do not stir now.
7. Scatter Parmesan cheese on top. Cover the skillet with a lid. Cook until it looks set around the edges. Turn off the heat.
8. In the meantime, set up your oven to broil mode. Place the rack 6 inches below the heating element—preheat the oven to high heat.
9. Shift the skillet into the oven and broil until it sets in the middle. It should take 7 – 10 minutes.
10. Remove the skillet from the oven and let it cool for 5 minutes. Cut into 4 equal wedges.
11. While the frittata is cooling, make the green juice by juicing together kale, parsley lettuce, ginger, apples, and celery in a juicer.
12. Add lemon juice and matcha green tea powder and stir.
13. Pour into 4 glasses and serve it along with frittata.

Buckwheat Blueberry Muffins with Coffee Smoothie

Preparation time: 10 minutes

Cooking time: 17 minutes
Number of servings: 5
Nutritional values per serving: 1 muffin with 1 smoothie

Muffin | Smoothie
Calories – 150 | Calories – 148
Fat – 8 g | Fat – 8.4 g
Carbohydrate – 17 g | Carbohydrate – 17 g
Protein – 3 g | Protein – 4.2 g

Ingredients:
For muffins, dry ingredients:

- ¼ cup buckwheat flour
- 1 tablespoon arrowroot flour
- 3 tablespoons almond flour
- ½ teaspoon baking powder
- 1 teaspoon coconut sugar
- ¼ teaspoon sea salt

For muffins, wet ingredients:

- 1 egg
- 1 tablespoon honey
- ½ cup blueberries, fresh or frozen +10 – 12 extra to top
- ½ small ripe banana, mashed
- 2 tablespoons butter, melted
- ¼ teaspoon vanilla extract

For muffins, streusel topping:

- ½ tablespoon sliced almonds

- ¼ tablespoon coconut sugar
- ¼ teaspoon ground cinnamon
- ¼ tablespoon buckwheat flour
- ¼ tablespoon butter, melted
- A tiny pinch sea salt

<u>For coffee smoothie:</u>

- 5 tablespoons ground coffee beans (do not use instant coffee)
- 2 ½ teaspoons vanilla extract
- 1 ¼ cups brewed coffee, chilled
- 5 tablespoons raw honey
- 4 ½ cups unsweetened almond milk
- 2 ½ ripe bananas, sliced, frozen
- Ice cubes, as required

Directions:

1. Preheat the oven to 350°F.
2. To make muffins: Add all the dry ingredients i.e., flours, coconut sugar, salt, and baking powder into a mixing bowl and stir well.
3. Add egg, honey, banana, and vanilla into another bowl and whisk until well combined. Pour this mixture into the bowl of dry ingredients and whisk until just combined, making sure not to over-mix.
4. Add blueberries and fold gently.
5. Grease 5 muffin cups with some olive oil cooking spray.
6. Divide the batter among the cups.
7. To make streusel topping: Add almond, sugar, buckwheat flour, cinnamon, butter, and salt into a

bowl and mix well. Scatter this mixture on top of the batter. Place 2 – 3 blueberries on top, in each muffin cup.
8. Place the muffin cups in an oven and bake for about 20 minutes. You can check it by inserting a toothpick in the center of the muffins. When you lift the toothpick out of the muffin, it should not have any particles stuck on it. If particles are stuck on it, bake for a few more minutes.
9. Once baked, remove the muffin cups from the oven and set aside to cool.
10. Run a knife around the edges of the muffins to loosen the muffins. Remove onto a plate.
11. Few minutes before serving, make the smoothie. For this, add ground coffee, brewed coffee, milk, ice cubes, vanilla, honey, and banana into a blender.
12. Blitz until very smooth.
13. Pour into 5 glasses and serve along with muffins.

Ultimate Tofu Breakfast Burrito Bowls

Preparation time: 15 minutes
Cooking time: 30 minutes
Number of servings: 2

Nutritional values per serving:
Calories – 579.2
Fat – 39.6 g
Carbohydrate – 59.2 g
Protein – 22 g

Ingredients:

For tofu scramble:

- 2 tablespoons olive oil
- Salt to taste
- 9.4 ounces extra-firm tofu, drained, cubed
- Pepper to taste
- 1 teaspoon garlic powder
- 1 teaspoon onion powder
- 2 teaspoons fresh lemon juice

For beans:

- 2/3 cup finely diced red onion
- ¾ tablespoon olive oil
- Salt to taste
- ¼ teaspoon turmeric powder
- 1 jalapeño pepper, deseeded, chopped
- 2 cloves garlic, peeled, minced
- 1 teaspoon ground cumin
- 1 1/3 cups chopped tomatoes
- A handful fresh cilantro, chopped
- 2/3 can (from a 15.5 ounces can) black beans, drained, rinsed

To serve:

- 1 cup cooked hash brown potatoes
- Lemon juice to drizzle
- 2/3 avocado, peeled, pitted, sliced
- Hot sauce to taste
- A handful fresh cilantro, chopped

Directions:

1. Place a heavy skillet over medium-high flame. Add 1 ½ tablespoons of oil. Once the oil is heated, add tofu, salt, and pepper and cook until brown. Stir often.
2. Stir in turmeric powder, garlic powder, and onion powder—cook for a couple of minutes.
3. Add ½ tablespoon oil and lemon juice and mix well. Turn off the heat after 5 minutes. Stir frequently during this time.
4. To make beans: Place another pan over medium-high heat. It is better to place a heavy-bottomed pan.
5. Pour oil into it. When the oil is heated, add onion, salt, and jalapeños and cook until onion turns pink.
6. Stir in garlic and sauté for a few seconds until you get a nice aroma in the air.
7. Stir in cumin and tomatoes. Add some salt to taste. Cook until tomatoes are soft.
8. Stir in lemon juice and cilantro—cook for a couple of minutes.
9. Stir in the beans and heat thoroughly, stirring often.
10. To assemble: Divide hash browns into 2 serving bowls. Divide the beans into the bowls and place it over the hash browns.
11. Scatter avocado on top. Drizzle lemon juice and hot sauce on top. Garnish with cilantro and serve.

Smoked Salmon Eggs Benedict with Iced Coffee

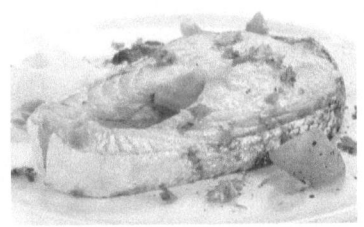

Preparation time: 35 minutes
Cooking time: 5 minutes
Number of servings: 4
Nutritional values per serving:

Egg benedict | Iced coffee
Calories – 388 | Calories – 28
Fat – 17.2 g | Fat – 1.3 g
Carbohydrate – 31.5 g | Carbohydrate – 1 g
Protein – 350 g | Protein – 0.6 g

Ingredients:
For smoked salmon egg benedict:

- 8 large eggs
- ½ cup cream cheese
- 4 teaspoons capers
- Pepper to taste
- 4 English muffins, split
- 6 ounces smoked salmon
- 1 red onion, thinly sliced

For the lemon-hollandaise sauce:

- 4 large egg yolks
- ¼ cup butter
- Salt to taste
- 4 tablespoons water
- 4 teaspoons fresh lemon juice

<u>For iced coffee:</u>

- 1 cup cold, brewed coffee
- Ice cubes, as required
- 1 cup milk of your choice
- 2 teaspoons vanilla extract

Directions:

1. To make hollandaise sauce: Combine yolks and water in a pan.
2. Turn on the flame of the gas stove to a medium-high flame.
3. Hold the pan about 2 inches above the flame and constantly whisk until warm.
4. Whisk in the butter. Keep whisking until the sauce thickens. Make sure that at no time, the pan should be placed directly on the burner.
5. Add lemon juice and salt to taste and whisk well. Now place the pan on your countertop.
6. To poach eggs: Pour water into a saucepan and place the saucepan over a high flame.
7. As it starts boiling, lower the flame and break the eggs into the pot and poach the eggs for 4 minutes.
8. In the meantime, toast the muffins in a toaster to the desired crispiness. Spread cream cheese on the cut part of the muffins and spread an equal amount

of salmon on the bottom half of each of the muffins.
9. Remove the eggs from the pot and place an egg on top of the salmon. Cover with the top half of the muffins and serve with iced coffee.
10. To make iced coffee: Divide milk, coffee, and vanilla into 2 tall glasses. Stir well.
11. Add ice cubes and serve.

Kale Egg Breakfast Cups Recipe

Preparation time: 10 minutes
Cooking time: 35 minutes
Number of servings: 6
Nutritional values per serving: 1 cup

Calories – 146
Fat – 8 g
Carbohydrate – 10 g
Protein – 10 g

Ingredients:

- ½ tablespoon olive oil
- 2 cloves garlic, peeled, minced
- 4 ounces hot chicken sausage
- Salt to taste
- 1 cup chopped kale
- 3 eggs or ¾ cup egg substitute
- ½ medium red onion, finely chopped
- 4 ounces mushrooms, thinly sliced
- ½ ounce sun-dried tomatoes, finely chopped

- 4 ounces feta cheese, crumbled
- Pepper to taste

Directions:

1. Preheat the oven to 350°F.
2. Prepare 6 muffin cups by spraying with cooking spray.
3. Place a skillet over medium flame. Add oil. When the oil is heated, add onion and cook until it turns pink.
4. Stir in the garlic and cook for about a minute.
5. Stir in the mushrooms. Cook until slightly brown.
6. Stir in the sausage and cook until brown, breaking it simultaneously as it cooks.
7. Now add sundried tomatoes and kale and cook for a couple of minutes.
8. Remove the pan from heat. Add feta and mix well.
9. Divide the mixture into the prepared muffin cups.
10. Add one beaten egg into each muffin cup. Add salt and pepper to taste and stir lightly.
11. Place the muffin cups in an oven and bake for about about 25 – 30 minutes. You can check it by inserting a toothpick in the center of the muffins. When you lift the toothpick out of the muffin, it should not have any particles stuck on it. If particles are stuck on it, bake for a few more minutes.
12. Once baked, remove the muffin cups from the oven and set aside to cool for a few minutes.
13. Remove the muffins from the cup.
14. Serve warm.

CHAPTER 5
LUNCH RECIPES

Kale, Quinoa, and Avocado Salad with Lemon Dijon Vinaigrette

Preparation time: 25 minutes
Cooking time: 15 minutes
Number of servings: 2

Nutritional values per serving:
Calories – 342.5
Fat – 20.3 g
Carbohydrate – 35.4 g
Protein – 8.9 g

Ingredients:
For salad:

- 1/3 cup quinoa
- ½ bunch kale, discard hard stems and ribs, torn
- ¼ cup chopped cucumber

- 1 tablespoon chopped red onion
- 2/3 cup water
- ¼ avocado, peeled, pitted, diced
- 3 tablespoons chopped red bell pepper
- ½ tablespoon crumbled feta cheese

For dressing:

- 2 tablespoons olive oil
- ¾ tablespoon Dijon mustard
- Pepper to taste
- 1 tablespoon lemon juice
- Salt to taste

Directions:

1. To cook quinoa: Add quinoa and water into a saucepan. Place the saucepan over medium-high heat. Once it begins to boil, lower the heat to medium-low and cook covered until dry. Turn off the heat and let it cool.
2. In the meantime, steam the kale. For this pour an inch of water into the pan. Place the saucepan over medium flame. Once it begins to boil, place a steamer basket with kale in the saucepan.
3. Cover and cook for 45 – 60 seconds. Spread kale on a serving platter.
4. Fluff quinoa with a fork and spread it over the kale. Scatter bell pepper, avocado, onion, cucumber, and feta cheese on top.
5. To make the dressing: Add oil, Dijon mustard, pepper, lemon juice, and salt into a bowl.
6. Whisk until emulsified.

7. Spoon the dressing over the salad and serve.

Kale Salad with Apples and Chicken

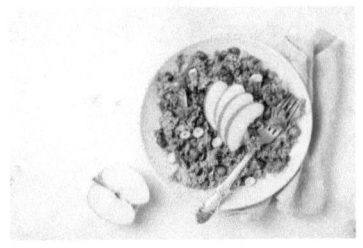

Preparation time: 10 minutes
Cooking time: 20 minutes
Number of servings: 2

Nutritional values per serving:
Calories – 362
Fat – 21 g
Carbohydrate – 28 g
Protein – 19 g

Ingredients:
For salad:

- 2 ½ cups chopped kale, discard hard stems and ribs
- ½ apple, cored, diced
- 2 tablespoons raisins
- 2 tablespoons chopped walnuts
- ¾ cup cooked, shredded chicken
- 2 tablespoons dried cherries
- 1 small red onion, thinly sliced

For apple cider vinaigrette:

- 3 tablespoons extra-virgin olive oil
- ½ tablespoon honey
- Salt to taste
- 2 small cloves garlic, peeled, minced
- 2 tablespoons apple cider vinegar
- ¼ teaspoon Dijon mustard
- Pepper to taste

Directions:

1. To make the dressing: Add oil, honey, salt, garlic, vinegar, mustard, and pepper into a small jar.
2. Tighten the lid and shake vigorously until well combined. Set aside for a while for the flavors to meld.
3. Place kale in a serving bowl. Add chicken, dried cherries, onion, apple, raisins, and walnuts and toss well.
4. Pour apple cider vinaigrette over it. Toss well.
5. Divide equally into 2 plates and serve.

Chicken & Vegetable Penne with Parsley-Walnut Pesto

Preparation time: 10 minutes
Cooking time: 20 minutes
Number of servings: 2
Nutritional values per serving: ½ the recipe

Calories – 514
Fat – 26.6 g
Carbohydrate – 43.4 g
Protein – 31.4 g

Ingredients:

- 1/3 cup chopped walnuts
- 1 clove garlic, peeled
- Pepper to taste
- 3 tablespoons grated parmesan cheese
- 3 ounces whole-wheat penne or fusilli pasta
- 4 ounces cauliflower florets
- ½ cup parsley leaves
- Salt to taste
- 1 tablespoon extra-virgin olive oil
- 4 ounces shredded or chopped chicken breasts
- 4 ounces green beans, halved crosswise

Directions:

1. Half fill a pot with water and place it over high heat. When it comes to a boil, add pasta and boil for 4 minutes.
2. Add cauliflower and green beans. Once pasta is al dente, drain it in a colander. Retain about ½ cup of the cooked pasta water.
3. While the pasta is cooking, add walnuts into a microwave-safe bowl and cook on high in a microwave until it is toasted lightly. You can also toast them in a skillet over a medium-low flame.
4. Let the walnuts cool completely. Retain a few walnuts pieces for garnishing. Use remaining walnuts to make pesto.
5. To make pesto: Add walnuts, garlic, parsley, pepper, and salt into a blender and blend until well combined.

6. With the blender machine running, pour oil and blend until smooth.
7. Add Parmesan cheese and blend until well combined.
8. Transfer the pesto into a bowl. Add chicken and some of the retained cooking water. Mix well.
9. Add pasta and toss well.
10. Serve garnished with retained walnuts.

Chicory, Sausage & Black Olive Polenta Tart

Preparation time: 10 minutes
Cooking time: 35 minutes
Number of servings: 2
Nutritional values per serving: ½ tart

Calories – 432
Fat – 33 g
Carbohydrate – 14 g
Protein – 19 g

Ingredients:

- Juice of ½ orange
- Zest of ½ orange, grated
- 1 – 2 heads red chicory, halved
- 3.5 ounces quick-cook polenta
- ½ vegetable or chicken stock cube
- 2 cups boiling water
- 3.5 ounces Taleggio cheese or mozzarella cheese, thinly sliced, chopped into small pieces
- 2 – 3 tablespoons pitted, halved black olives

- 2 Italian sausages, discard casing, crumbled
- 1 teaspoon honey
- Extra virgin olive oil, to drizzle
- Red chili flakes to taste
- Seasoning of your choice

Directions:

1. Preheat the oven to 350°F.
2. Add honey and orange juice into a pan and place the pan over a medium-low flame.
3. Simmer until slightly thick. Stir in chicory and cook for a couple of minutes. Turn the chicory half-way through cooking. Turn off the heat and let the chicory cool. As it cools, cut the chicory into 2 halves.
4. Prepare a baking sheet by lining it with parchment paper. Grease it with oil.
5. Add boiling water and stock cube into a pan. Place the pan over medium flame. Add polenta and cook until thick. Keep constantly whisking until very thick.
6. Turn off the heat and spread the mixture on the prepared baking sheet. It should be around 1 inch thick.
7. Scatter the cheese cubes over the polenta layer. Next lay the chicory pieces over the polenta layer. Now scatter sausage, orange zest, and olives over the chicory layer.
8. Sprinkle seasoning and red chili flakes on top. Drizzle the oil on top.
9. Place the baking sheet in the oven and bake for about 20 minutes.

10. Now set the oven to broil mode and broil for 4 – 5 minutes until sausage turns brown.
11. Remove the baking sheet from the oven and let it cool on your countertop for 15 minutes.
12. Cut into 2 halves.
13. Serve.

Lovage and Potato Soup

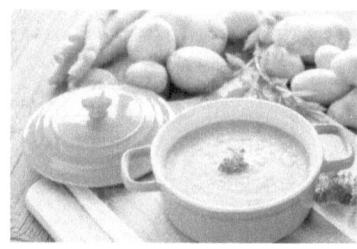

Preparation time: 20 minutes
Cooking time: 30 minutes
Number of servings: 8
Nutritional values per serving: 9.6 ounces

Calories – 316.6
Fat – 8.4 g
Carbohydrate – 52.5 g
Protein – 9.5 g

Ingredients:

- 2 medium onions, finely chopped
- 4.4 pounds potatoes, scrubbed, cubed
- 4 cups milk
- 1 cup chopped lovage
- Pepper to taste

- 2 tablespoons olive oil
- 4 cups vegetable or chicken stock
- Salt to taste

Directions:

1. Place a soup pot over medium flame. Add oil and let it heat. Cook the onions in the pot until pink.
2. Stir in the potatoes. Give it a good mix.
3. Pour stock and milk. As it starts boiling, lower the heat and cook covered until potatoes are soft. Turn off the heat. Blend the soup until smooth. Add more stock if you want to dilute the soup.
4. Taste and add salt and pepper to taste.

Kale Caesar Salad Bowls with Tofu Croutons

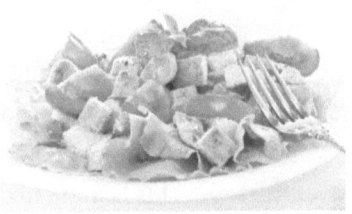

Preparation time: 40 minutes
Cooking time: 15 to 20 min minutes
Number of servings: 2

Nutritional values per serving:
Calories – 400
Fat – 28 g
Carbohydrate – 19 g
Protein – 20 g

Ingredients:

<u>For tofu croutons:</u>

- 7 ounces block extra-firm tofu, drained
- 2 tablespoons vegan Worcestershire sauce
- ½ teaspoon onion powder
- ½ teaspoon garlic powder
- 2 tablespoons lemon juice
- 1 ½ teaspoon olive oil

<u>For salad bowl:</u>

- 4 cups chopped lacinato kale
- 2 tablespoons toasted pumpkin seeds
- ½ avocado, peeled, pitted chopped
- 2 tablespoons nutritional yeast
- ¼ cup bottled vegan Caesar dressing

Directions:

1. To make tofu croutons: Place a few sheets of paper towels on a plate. Place the tofu over it. Place a heavy pan over the tofu. This is done to drain excess moisture from the tofu.
2. Let it remain like this for 15 – 20 minutes.
3. Cut into ¾ inch cubes.
4. To make the dressing: Combine lemon juice, garlic powder, onion powder, and Worcestershire sauce in a bowl.
5. Add tofu and toss well. Cover and set aside for about 15 minutes.
6. Place a skillet over medium flame. Add oil and allow it to heat. Once the oil is heated, add only the

tofu into the pan and discard the marinade. Cook until tofu turns golden brown all over. Turn the tofu often until golden brown.

7. Remove the tofu with a slotted spoon and place on a plate lined with paper towels.
8. To assemble: Add kale into a bowl. Sprinkle nutritional yeast over it and toss well.
9. Divide kale into 2 bowls.
10. Place half the tofu croutons in each of the bowls. Sprinkle a tablespoon of pumpkin seeds in each bowl.
11. Scatter avocado on top.
12. Drizzle vegan Caesar salad dressing on top and serve.

CHAPTER 6
DINNER RECIPES

Cashew Buckwheat Curry with Garlic Kale

Preparation time: 15 minutes
Cooking time: 30 minutes
Number of servings: 6
Nutritional values per serving: 1/6 recipe (without optional serving options)

Calories – 474
Fat – 31.4 g
Carbohydrate – 45.5 g
Protein – 10.8 g

Ingredients:
For curry:

- 2 onions, finely chopped
- 2 tablespoons grated fresh ginger

- 1 ½ cups buckwheat groats
- 1 teaspoon ground cumin
- 2 teaspoons smoked paprika
- 2 teaspoons ground coriander
- 2 teaspoons turmeric powder
- 2 cans (14 ounces each) coconut milk
- ½ teaspoon sriracha sauce
- 3 cups finely chopped kale leaves, discard hard stems and ribs
- 4 cloves garlic, peeled, minced
- ½ cup cashews
- 2 tablespoons coconut sugar
- 4 tablespoons soy sauce
- 3 cups water or more if required
- 2 teaspoons lemon juice or to taste
- 2 tablespoons coconut oil

For garlic kale:

- 6 cups chopped kale, discard hard stems and ribs, cut into bite-size pieces
- 4 cloves garlic, peeled, minced
- Salt to taste
- 2 tablespoons olive oil
- Pepper to taste

To serve: Optional

- Hot steamed rice
- Cooked quinoa
- Flatbreads
- Naan bread
- Chapatti, etc.

Directions:

1. To make the curry: Place a large skillet over medium flame. Add oil and let it melt.
2. Once the oil has melted, add onion, ginger, and garlic and cook until it begins to become light brown. Stir frequently.
3. Stir in the cashews and buckwheat groats and cook until it turns brown, sort of golden brown. Stir frequently to avoid burning them.
4. Stir in turmeric and cook for 5 – 6 seconds. Next add coriander, paprika, cumin, and coconut sugar and mix well.
5. Add water, coconut milk, sriracha sauce, soy sauce, and kale and mix well.
6. As the mixture comes to a boil, lower the heat and cook covered until soft. Add more water if the curry is dry.
7. Turn off the heat. Add lemon juice and stir. Transfer into a bowl and keep warm.
8. In the meantime, make garlic kale. For this, place a skillet with oil over medium flame.
9. Once the oil is heated, add garlic and cook for a few seconds until garlic turns aromatic.
10. Stir in maple syrup and kale and cook until kale wilts.
11. Add salt and pepper to taste.
12. Transfer into a bowl.
13. Serve curry with garlic kale as it is or with any of the serving options.

Crispy Peanut Tofu & Cauliflower Rice Stir-Fry

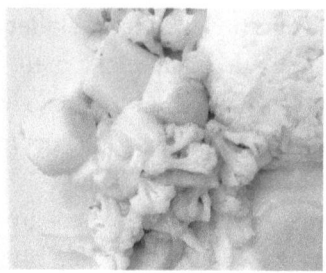

Preparation time: 30 minutes
Cooking time: 60 minutes
Number of servings: 4
Nutritional values per serving: ¼ of the recipe, without optional ingredients

Calories – 524
Fat – 24.5 g
Carbohydrate – 38.4 g
Protein – 24.5 g

Ingredients:
For stir-fry:

- 24 ounces extra-firm tofu
- 2 small heads cauliflower
- 2 tablespoons toasted sesame oil
- 4 cloves garlic, peeled, minced
- Baby Bok Choy, as required (optional)
- Red pepper, as required (optional)
- Green onions, as required (optional)
- Broccoli, as required (optional)

For sauce:

- 3 tablespoons toasted sesame oil
- ½ cup light brown sugar
- 5 tablespoons peanut butter or almond butter
- ½ cup low-sodium soy sauce
- 1 teaspoon chili garlic sauce

To serve:

- Lime juice
- Sriracha sauce
- Chopped cilantro
- Any other toppings of your choice

Directions:

1. Preheat the oven to 350°F.
2. Place a few sheets of paper towels on a plate and put the tofu over it. Place a heavy pan over the tofu. This is done to drain excess moisture from the tofu.
3. Let it remain like this for 20 minutes.
4. In the meantime, make the sauce. For this, combine sesame oil, sugar, peanut butter, soy sauce, and chili garlic sauce in a bowl. Whisk until well combined.
5. Once drained, cut the tofu into cubes.
6. Prepare a baking sheet by lining it with parchment paper. Spread the tofu on it, without overlapping.
7. Place the baking sheet in the oven and leave to dry for about 25 minutes.
8. Take out the baking sheet from the oven and let the tofu cool for 20 minutes. Add tofu into the bowl of sauce and mix well. Let it sit for 15 minutes.

9. To make cauliflower rice: Grate the cauliflower. You can do this in the food processor or grate it with the larger holes of a box grater. If using a food processor, cut the cauliflower into florets before adding it to the processor.
10. Chop the optional vegetables if using.
11. Place a large skillet over medium-high flame. Add a little of the sesame oil and let it heat. Add the optional vegetables if using along with soy sauce and cook until tender. Transfer into a bowl and keep warm.
12. Add only tofu from the sauce into the pan, using a slotted spoon. Cook until brown. It will stick to the pan because of the sauce.
13. Transfer the tofu into a bowl.
14. Clean the pan and place the pan over medium flame. Add remaining oil and let it heat.
15. Add garlic and grated cauliflower and mix well. Cook covered for about 5 minutes or until tender and light brown.
16. Add 1 – 2 tablespoons of sauce mixture or enough to suit your taste and mix well.
17. Divide cauliflower rice into serving plates.
18. Place tofu and cooked vegetables on top. Drizzle remaining sauce mixture on top if desired and serve.

Steak, Asparagus & Walnut Stir-Fry with Creamy Au Gratin Potatoes

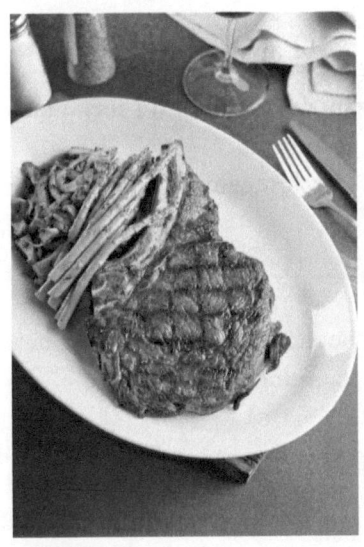

Preparation time: 30 minutes
Cooking time: 1 hour and 20 minutes
Number of servings: 2
Nutritional values per serving:

Au gratin potatoes | Steak stir fry
Calories – 498.8 | Calories – 442
Fat – 25.4 g | Fat – 23 g
Carbohydrate – 49.3 g | Carbohydrate – 24 g
Protein – 19.8 g | Protein – 36 g

Ingredients:

- ½ pound beef strip steaks, boneless (¾ inch thick), cut into ¼ inch strips, across the grain

- ½ tablespoon olive oil, divided
- ¼ cup walnut halves
- Salt to taste
- ¼ cup crumbled blue cheese
- ½ cup uncooked instant brown rice
- ½ pound asparagus, cut into 2-inch pieces
- 1 clove garlic, minced
- ¼ cup fat- free, low sodium beef broth

For creamy au gratin potatoes:

- 2 medium potatoes (about 3-inch diameter), cut into ¼ inch thick, round slices
- Salt to taste
- 1 ½ tablespoon all-purpose flour
- 1 cup milk
- Pepper to taste
- 1 medium onion, cut into round slices
- 1 ½ tablespoons butter
- ¾ cup shredded cheddar cheese

Directions:

1. Preheat the oven to 400°F.
2. Start by making the creamy au gratin potatoes, as it will take time to bake.
3. Take a small casserole dish and grease it with some butter.
4. Spread half the potato slices in the dish. Layer with onion slices followed by the rest of the potatoes.
5. Sprinkle salt and pepper on each layer.
6. Place a small saucepan over medium flame. Add

butter. Once butter melts, add flour and keep stirring for a minute.

7. Add milk and continue stirring until thick. Add cheese and mix well. Turn off the heat after cheese melts.
8. Spoon the cheese sauce over the potatoes. Keep the dish covered with foil and place the casserole dish in the oven and bake for about 1 hour and 20 minutes for the potatoes to cook.
9. Meanwhile, follow the instructions on the package and cook the brown rice. Once the rice is cooked, keep it warm.
10. Cook the steak for 15 minutes before the baking time is over.
11. To cook steak: Place a large nonstick skillet over medium-high flame. Add ½ teaspoon oil and let it heat.
12. Add asparagus and sauté until crisp as well as tender.
13. Stir in the walnuts, salt, and garlic. Cook for a minute, stirring constantly. Transfer into a bowl and keep it warm.
14. Add remaining oil into the skillet. Add steak strips and cook until it is not pink anymore.
15. Add asparagus mixture and broth and mix well. Bring to a boil and turn off the heat.
16. Divide rice into 2 serving plates. Divide the steak slices and place over the rice. Sprinkle blue cheese on top and serve.

Garlic Parsley Chicken with Mashed Potatoes

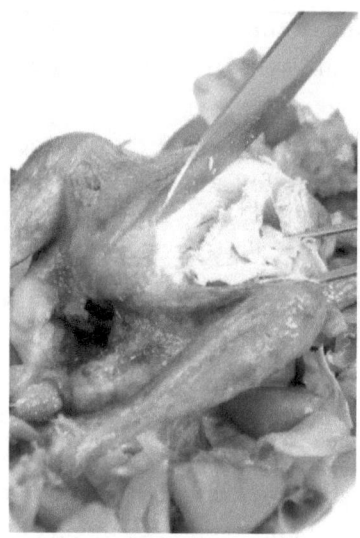

Preparation time: 20 minutes
Cooking time: 20 minutes
Number of servings: 3

Nutritional values per serving:
Garlic chicken | Mashed potatoes
Calories – 369 | Calories – 718
Fat – 20 g | Fat – 13.3 g
Carbohydrate – 17 g | Carbohydrate – 137.2 g
Protein – 29 g | Protein – 17.2 g

Ingredients:
For garlic parsley chicken:

- ½ pound boneless, skinless chicken breasts, thinly sliced

- 1 ½ tablespoon olive oil
- 4 cloves garlic, peeled, minced
- ½ large tomato, deseeded, diced
- 1 tablespoon butter
- Salt to taste
- ¼ cup flour
- Freshly ground pepper to taste
- 3 tablespoons chopped fresh parsley
- 1 cup sliced fresh mushrooms
- ¼ cup chicken stock
- ½ tablespoon grated parmesan cheese

For mashed potatoes:

- 1 pound small golden potatoes
- 1/3 cup whole milk
- 2 tablespoons chopped, fresh parsley
- Freshly ground pepper to taste
- 1 ½ tablespoon unsalted butter
- 5 cloves garlic, peeled, minced
- Salt to taste

Directions:

1. Start by making the mashed potatoes. For this, place the potatoes in a saucepan. Pour enough water to cover the potatoes. Add ½ teaspoon salt. Place the saucepan over medium flame. Once it begins to boil, lower the heat slightly and cook until potatoes are soft.
2. While the potatoes are boiling, make garlic parsley chicken: Place chicken on a plate. Sprinkle flour all over the chicken.

3. Place a skillet over medium-high flame. Add a tablespoon of oil and let it heat. Once the oil is hot, add chicken and cook until the underside is brown. Turn the chicken over and cook the other side for 5 minutes or until brown.
4. Transfer the chicken onto a plate.
5. Add ½ tablespoon oil into the skillet. Once the oil is heated, stir in the mushrooms. Stir continuously for about 3 minutes or until brown.
6. Pour stock and scrape the bottom of the pan to remove any particles that may be stuck.
7. Stir in tomato, parsley, garlic, butter, and cheese.
8. As the butter melts, add the chicken back into the pan. Heat thoroughly.
9. Turn off the heat and keep warm.
10. Drain the water from the saucepan of potatoes. Blend the potatoes with an immersion blender until smooth. You can mash it if you do not like a smooth texture.
11. Add milk and butter and mix well.
12. Add parsley, garlic, pepper, and salt and mix well.
13. Serve chicken with mashed potatoes.

Tempeh Fajitas

Preparation time: 30 minutes
Cooking time: 5 minutes
Number of servings: 2
Nutritional values per serving: 1 fajita

Calories – 259
Fat – 5.1 g

Carbohydrate – 47.3 g
Protein – 14.6 g

Ingredients:
For filling:

- ½ package (from an 8 ounces package) five-grain tempeh, cut into 6 strips
- 2 tablespoons low-sodium soy sauce
- 1 teaspoon ground cumin
- Freshly ground pepper to taste
- 1 cup sliced red onions
- ½ cup pineapple juice
- 1 tablespoon fresh lime juice
- 1 teaspoon canola oil
- 2 small cloves garlic, peeled, minced
- ¾ cup sliced green bell peppers (½ inch thick)
- Salt to taste

To serve:

- 2 tablespoons chipotle salsa
- 2 whole-wheat tortillas (8 inches each)

Directions:

1. Add pineapple juice, lime juice, oil, garlic, cumin, soy sauce, and pepper into a saucepan and place the saucepan over medium flame.
2. When it begins to boil, turn off the heat.
3. Add tempeh into it and stir until well coated. Set aside on your countertop for 30 minutes.
4. Set up your grill and preheat it to medium heat.

5. Spray a wire-grilling basket with cooking spray.
6. Add onion and bell pepper into the grilling basket. Season with the salt and pepper, spray some cooking spray, and toss well.
7. Keep the grill basket on the grill rack. Turn occasionally until the onion turns light brown.
8. Remove the basket and set it aside.
9. Spray the grill rack with cooking spray.
10. Take out the tempeh from the saucepan and place it on the grill rack. Retain the marinade.
11. Lay the tempeh strips on the grill rack. Turn sides after grilling for 2 minutes, and baste the tempeh with the retained marinade while grilling.
12. Heat the tortillas following the directions on the package.
13. Place 3 tempeh strips on each tortilla and scatter half the onion mixture on each tortilla. Drizzle a tablespoon of salsa on each.
14. Roll and place with its seam side facing down. Cut into 2 halves if desired.
15. Serve.

Sesame Noodles with Baked Tofu

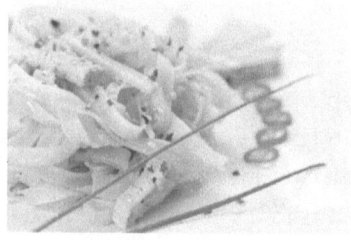

Preparation time: 10 minutes
Cooking time: 30 minutes
Number of servings: 2
Nutritional values per serving: 1-¾ cups

Calories – 458
Fat – 18 g
Carbohydrate – 60 g
Protein – 18 g

Ingredients:

- 4 ounces buckwheat noodles
- 1 scallion, chopped
- 1 teaspoon minced ginger
- 1 tablespoon low-sodium soy sauce
- 1 cup small broccoli florets
- 1 ½ tablespoon toasted peanuts
- 1 ½ tablespoon toasted dark sesame oil
- ½ tablespoon minced garlic
- ½ teaspoon brown sugar
- 1 tablespoon hoisin sauce
- 4 ounces tofu, cubed, baked
- ½ cups sliced yellow or orange bell pepper

Directions:

1. Follow the instructions on the package of pasta and cook the pasta. Place the cooked pasta in a bowl.
2. Place a saucepan over medium flame. Add oil, ginger, garlic, scallions, broccoli, and brown sugar. When the mixture is well heated, turn off the heat.

3. Add soy sauce and hoisin sauce. Transfer into the bowl of noodles.
4. Add tofu, peanuts, and bell pepper and toss well.
5. Serve.

CHAPTER 7
SNACK RECIPES

Baked Salmon Cake Balls with Rosemary Aioli

Preparation time: 5 minutes
Cooking time: 40 minutes
Number of servings: 6
Nutritional values per serving: 2 balls with 1 tablespoon aioli

Calories – 173
Fat – 6.7 g
Carbohydrate – 8.6 g
Protein – 20.5 g

Ingredients:
For salmon cake balls:

- 1 pound wild salmon fillets
- Pepper to taste
- ¼ yellow bell pepper, chopped
- ¼ red bell pepper chopped

- 1/3 cup breadcrumbs
- ¼ cup chopped parsley
- ¼ cup chopped spinach
- ¼ cup Dijon mustard
- 2 tablespoons lemon juice
- ¼ cup vegan mayonnaise
- 1 small egg, at room temperature
- 1 tablespoon sriracha sauce
- 2 tablespoons fresh lemon juice
- Salt to taste
- 1 small red onion, chopped
- ½ jalapeño, diced
- ½ - 1 tablespoon Old Bay seasoning

<u>For rosemary aioli</u>

- ¼ cup vegan mayonnaise
- 1 clove garlic, peeled, crushed, minced
- 1 sprig rosemary, chopped
- Salt to taste
- 1 tablespoon fresh lemon juice

Directions:

1. Preheat the oven to 400°F.
2. Prepare a baking sheet by lining it with parchment paper.
3. Sprinkle salt and pepper all over the salmon and place it on the baking sheet.
4. Place the baking sheet in the oven and roast until it flakes readily when pierced with a fork. It should take around 20 minutes.
5. Take out the baking sheet from the oven and let it

cool for 5 minutes.
6. Shred the salmon into bite-size chunks.
7. Combine onion, jalapeño, Old Bay seasoning, parsley, egg, lemon juice, sriracha sauce, red bell pepper, yellow bell pepper, spinach, breadcrumbs, vegan mayonnaise, and Dijon mustard in a bowl.
8. Mix in the salmon until well combined.
9. Divide the mixture into 12 equal portions and shape into balls.
10. Place it on the baking sheet.
11. Bake for around 20 minutes or until golden brown.
12. Meanwhile, make the aioli by combining vegan mayonnaise, garlic, rosemary, salt, and lemon juice in a bowl.
13. Serve salmon balls with aioli.

Healthy Coffee Cookies

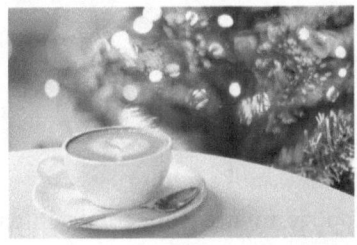

Preparation time: 15 – 20 minutes
Cooking time: 12 - 15 minutes
Number of servings: 20
Nutritional values per serving: 1 cookie

Calories – 60
Fat – 1.5 g
Carbohydrate – 11 g

Protein – 2 g

Ingredients:
For dry ingredients:

- ½ cup cocoa, unsweetened
- 6 tablespoons all-purpose flour
- ½ cup whole-wheat flour
- ¾ tablespoon finely ground coffee beans or instant coffee
- ½ teaspoon baking soda
- ¾ teaspoon ground cinnamon
- ¼ teaspoon kosher salt

For wet ingredients:

- 3 small eggs, lightly beaten
- ¼ cup nonfat or low-fat plain Greek yogurt
- ½ tablespoon olive oil
- ½ + 1/8 cup blueberries
- ½ ripe banana
- ¼ cup honey
- 1 teaspoon pure vanilla extract
- ¼ cup dark or semi-sweet chocolate chips

Directions:

1. Preheat the oven to 350°F.
2. Prepare a baking sheet by spraying with nonstick cooking spray. Set it aside.
3. Combine all the dry ingredients i.e. whole-wheat flour, all-purpose flour, cocoa, cinnamon, salt, baking soda, and coffee in a mixing bowl.

4. Place banana in a microwave-safe bowl and cook on high for about 50 seconds.
5. Mash the banana and add into a bowl. Also add eggs, yogurt, oil, honey, and vanilla. Mix until well incorporated.
6. Pour the wet ingredients into the dry ingredients and mix until just combined, making sure not to over-mix.
7. Add chocolate chips and blueberries and fold gently.
8. Make 20 equal portions of the mixture and place it on the baking sheet. It should be approximately 1-½ tablespoons per portion.
9. Press the cookies lightly. You can use a fork to do so.
10. Place the baking sheet in the oven and bake for about 12 – 14 minutes. When the cookies are ready, they will be visibly hard around the edges.
11. Cool on the baking sheet for 10 minutes. Loosen the cookies by pushing a metal spatula underneath the cookies. Transfer onto a wire rack
12. Let it cool completely before transferring into an airtight container.

Healthy Strawberry Oatmeal Bars

Preparation time: 20 minutes
Cooking time: 35 – 40 minutes
Number of servings: 8
Nutritional values per serving: 1 bar without glaze

Calories – 100
Fat – 5 g

Carbohydrate – 14 g
Protein – 2 g

Ingredients:
For strawberry bars:

- ½ cup old-fashioned rolled oats
- 3 tablespoons light brown sugar
- 1/8 teaspoon kosher salt
- 1 cup small-diced strawberries, divided
- ½ tablespoon fresh lemon juice
- 6 tablespoons white whole wheat flour
- 1/8 teaspoon ground ginger
- 3 tablespoons unsalted butter, melted
- ½ teaspoon cornstarch
- 3 teaspoons granulated sugar, divided

For the vanilla glaze: Optional

- ¼ cup powdered sugar, sifted
- ½ tablespoon milk
- ¼ teaspoon pure vanilla extract

Directions:

1. Preheat the oven to 350°F.
2. Set the rack in the center of the oven.
3. Prepare a small square or rectangular baking pan by lining it with a large sheet of parchment paper such that the extra sheet is hanging from 2 opposite sides.
4. Add oats, brown sugar, flour, salt, and ginger into a bowl and stir well.

5. Add butter and mix until well combined and sort of crumbly.
6. Take out about 4 tablespoons of the mixture into a bowl and set it aside.
7. Transfer the rest of the mixture into the baking pan. Press it well onto the bottom of the baking pan.
8. Spread ½ cup chopped strawberries over the crust —dust cornstarch over it.
9. Drizzle lemon juice over the strawberries. Sprinkle 1 ½ teaspoons sugar.
10. Spread remaining strawberries and 1 ½ teaspoons sugar over it.
11. Scatter the retained crumb mixture on top.
12. Place the baking dish in the oven and bake for about 30 – 35 minutes or until golden brown on top.
13. Take out the baking dish and place it on the wire rack to cool.
14. Meanwhile, make the glaze. For this, add powdered sugar, milk, and vanilla into a bowl and whisk well.
15. Lift the bars along with the parchment paper and place it on your cutting board.
16. Pour glaze on top. Cut into 8 equal bars and serve.
17. Place leftover bars in an airtight container. Place it in the refrigerator until use. It can last for 5 days.

Parsley Cheese Balls

Preparation time: 15 minutes
Cooking time: 0 minutes
Number of servings: 12
Nutritional values per serving: 1 cheese ball + 2 pieces celery + 5 crackers

Calories – 130
Fat – 7 g
Carbohydrate – 12 g
Protein – 3 g

Ingredients:

- ¼ cup shredded, Kraft 2% milk sharp cheddar cheese
- 1 package (8 ounces) Philadelphia Neufchatel cheese, softened
- ½ tablespoon finely chopped green onion
- ½ tablespoon finely chopped red pepper
- ¼ cup finely chopped parsley
- 1 teaspoon Dijon mustard
- 6 stalks celery, cut each into 4 equal pieces crosswise
- 60 whole-wheat Ritz crackers

Directions:

1. Add Neufchatel and cheddar cheeses into a bowl. Beat with an electric hand mixer until well combined.
2. Stir in green onion, red pepper, and Dijon mustard.
3. Place the bowl in the refrigerator for an hour.
4. Divide the mixture into 12 equal portions and shape into balls. (It should be 2 tablespoons cheese mixture per portion)
5. Place parsley on a plate. Dredge the balls in parsley.
6. Place on a plate. Chill until use.
7. To serve: Each serving should consist of a cheese ball with 2 pieces parsley and 5 Ritz crackers.

Baked Kale Chips

Preparation time: 10 minutes
Cooking time: 10 minutes
Number of servings: 3

Nutritional values per serving:
Calories – 58
Fat – 2.8 g
Carbohydrate – 7.6 g
Protein – 2.5 g

Ingredients:

- ½ bunch kale (hard stems and ribs discarded), torn into bite-size pieces
- Salt to taste
- ½ tablespoon olive oil
- Spices of your choice to taste (optional)

Directions:

1. Preheat the oven to 350°F.
2. Prepare a baking sheet by lining it with parchment paper.
3. Dry the kale using a salad spinner. If you do not have a salad spinner, pat the leaves dry with paper towels.
4. Place kale on the baking sheet. Trickle oil over it. Sprinkle salt over the kale and spread it evenly.
5. Place the baking sheet in the oven and bake for about 12 – 14 minutes or until crisp.

6. Cool completely and serve. Store the leftovers in an airtight container.

CHAPTER 8
DESSERT RECIPES

Chocolate Covered Date with Almonds

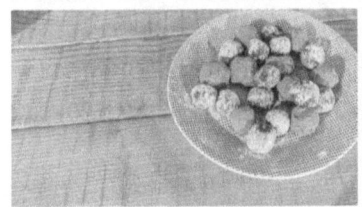

Preparation time: 20 minutes
Cooking time: 5 minutes
Nutritional values per serving: 12

Calories – 152
Fat – 5.4 g
Carbohydrate – 27.5 g
Protein – 2 g

Ingredients:

- 12 Medjool dates (slitted, with pit removed)

- ¾ cup semi-sweet chocolate chips
- ½ teaspoon ground cinnamon
- 12 unsalted roasted almonds
- ½ teaspoon canola oil
- 1 teaspoon crushed almonds
- 1 teaspoon crushed pistachios

Directions:

1. Insert an almond in each date. The dates should completely cover the almond. Place them on a tray that has been lined with parchment paper.
2. Add cinnamon, canola oil, and chocolate chips into a heatproof bowl. Place the bowl in a double boiler. For setting a double boiler, pour some water into a pot. The heatproof bowl should just fit on the top of the pot. Place the pot over medium flame. The chocolate will slowly melt. Stir often until chocolate melts.
3. Turn off the heat and take out the heatproof bowl from the double boiler.
4. Dunk the almond stuffed date in the melted chocolate, one at a time. Lift it out with a spoon and place it back on the tray.
5. Mix pistachios and almonds in a small bowl.
6. Sprinkle almond and pistachios on the chocolate-coated dates. Place the tray in the freezer and freeze until the chocolate sets, about an hour.
7. Take out the tray from the freezer and place it on your countertop for 10 minutes before serving.
8. Serve.
9. Store leftovers in an airtight container in the refrigerator.

Vegan Matcha Swirl Cheesecake

Preparation time: 1 hour plus an additional 60 minutes
Cooking time: 0 minutes
Number of servings: 5
Nutritional values per serving: 1 slice, without optional toppings

Calories – 340
Fat – 23.5 g
Carbohydrate – 31.3 g
Protein – 7.3 g

Ingredients:
For filling:

- ¾ cup raw cashews
- 1 ½ tablespoon fresh lemon juice
- 2 tablespoons melted coconut oil
- 2 tablespoons coconut yogurt
- 1 teaspoon matcha green tea powder
- ¼ cup maple syrup
- 1/8 teaspoon sea salt
- ½ teaspoon vanilla extract
- 2 tablespoons light coconut milk

For the crust:

- ½ cup packed, pitted Medjool dates
- A wee bit sea salt
- ¾ cup walnuts

For the topping: Optional

- Fresh blueberries or strawberries
- Coconut whipped cream

Directions:

1. Place cashews in a bowl. Pour very hot water over it. Cover and set aside for an hour.
2. Discard the water.
3. While the cashews are soaking, make the crust: Take a small springform pan of about 5 – 6 inches diameter. Line it with parchment paper and set it aside.
4. Place dates in the food processor bowl and process until finely chopped. Transfer into a bowl.
5. Add walnuts and salt and blend until smooth. Add dates and process until the mixture comes together. When you press the mixture, it should not crumble and fall apart.
6. Transfer the mixture into the prepared springform pan. Press it well onto the bottom as well as a little on the sides of the dish.
7. Freeze the dish until the crust is slightly hard.
8. To make the filling: Add cashews, lemon juice, coconut oil, coconut yogurt, maple syrup, salt, vanilla, and coconut milk into a blender and blend until smooth in texture.
9. Set aside about 1/3 of the filling in the blender itself and spread the remaining on the crust. Tap the springform pan on your countertop lightly to remove air pockets if any.
10. Add matcha powder into the blender and blend

until smooth. Taste and add more matcha powder if desired.

11. Pour the matcha filling on top of the plain filling in a spiraling manner.
12. Using a chopstick or toothpick, swirl the matcha filling lightly into the plain filling.
13. Tap the springform pan once again, on your countertop lightly to remove air pockets if any.
14. Keep the pan covered loosely, with cling wrap. Place the pan in the freezer until set. It should feel firm when you touch it.
15. Remove from the freezer and refrigerate until use. It can last for 3 days.
16. 15 minutes before serving, place the pan in the freezer once again.
17. Cut into 5 equal wedges. Remove the springform pan.
18. Serve chilled.

Sticky Date and Walnut Pudding

Preparation time: 25 minutes
Cooking time: 60 minutes
Number of servings: 4

Nutritional values per serving:
Calories – 282
Fat – 16 g
Carbohydrate – 55 g
Protein – 6 g

Ingredients:

- ½ cup chopped dried, pitted dates
- ¼ cup reduced-salt margarine
- 1 egg, lightly beaten
- 1/8 teaspoon ground cinnamon
- ¼ cup chopped, toasted walnuts
- 2 tablespoons low-fat milk
- ¼ cup brown sugar
- ½ cup self-rising flour
- ¼ teaspoon ground ginger

For pineapple and marmalade sauce:

- ½ can (from a 14.1 ounces can) pineapple in natural juice, finely chopped
- 2 ½ tablespoons fine cut orange marmalade
- ½ teaspoon arrowroot

Directions:

1. Preheat the oven to 350°F.
2. Prepare a small pudding basin by lining it with parchment paper (cut into a circle to fit the bottom of the basin).
3. Add dates and a tablespoon of milk into a bowl and stir well. Set aside.
4. Add sugar, margarine, a tablespoon of milk and egg into another bowl and whisk well.
5. Add flour, ground ginger, and cinnamon into a third bowl and stir well.
6. Add the flour mixture into the bowl of egg mixture and beat until smooth. You can use an electric hand mixer for this.
7. Add walnuts and the soaked dates and fold gently.

8. Pour the mixture into the pudding basin.
9. Place the pudding basin in a baking pan. Take some boiling water and pour it all around the pudding basin up to ½ inch.
10. Tent the baking pan as well as the pudding basin with foil.
11. Place the baking pan and the pudding basin, in the oven. Bake for about 50 minutes or until a toothpick inserted in the middle comes out clean. If it isn't clean, bake for another 10 minutes.
12. Take out the baking dish and place it on the wire rack to cool.
13. While the pudding is baking, make the pineapple and marmalade sauce. Use most of the juice of the pineapple (about 2/3). The rest can be used in some other recipe like a smoothie.
14. Add arrowroot and about a teaspoon of the pineapple juice in a small saucepan. Whisk well.
15. Add the rest of the juice and place the saucepan over medium flame. Bring to a boil, stirring constantly. It will be slightly thick.
16. Add pineapple pieces and marmalade. Stir well. Let it cook on low heat for a couple of minutes. Stir occasionally. Turn off the heat.
17. Invert the pudding onto a plate. Spread some of the sauce over it.
18. Cut into 4 equal portions and serve with some of the remaining sauce. It can be served warm or at room temperature.

Healthy Chocolate Pudding

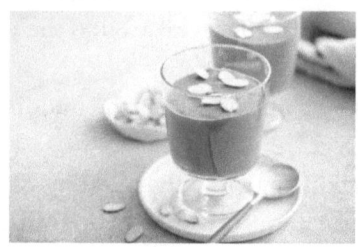

Preparation time: 5 minutes
Cooking time: 0 minutes
Number of servings: 4

Nutritional values per serving:
Calories – 454
Fat – 18 g
Carbohydrate – 69 g
Protein – 11 g

Ingredients:

- 2 ripe bananas, sliced
- ½ cup peanut butter
- ½ cup oats
- 1/8 teaspoon salt
- ½ cup cocoa powder
- ½ cup honey
- 1 teaspoon vanilla extract

Directions:

1. Blend bananas, peanut butter, oats, salt, cocoa, honey, and vanilla in a blender until smooth.

2. Divide equally into 4 dessert bowls. Cover the bowls with cling wrap.
3. Refrigerate for a couple of hours or until it sets.
4. Serve chilled.

Layered Frozen Chocolate Coffee Pops

Preparation time: 20 minutes
Cooking time: 0 minutes
Number of servings: 4

Nutritional values per serving:
Calories – 78
Fat – 0.4 g
Carbohydrate – 16.2 g
Protein – 3.2 g

Ingredients:

- ½ package (from a 4 serving size package) fat- free, sugar-free, low calorie white instant chocolate pudding mix
- 1 cup fat-free milk
- 3 tablespoons fat-free sweetened condensed milk
- 1 teaspoon instant espresso coffee powder or more to taste
- ¾ cup water
- 2 tablespoons cocoa powder, unsweetened
- ¼ teaspoon vanilla extract

Directions:

1. For the first layer: Add pudding mix, ¾ teaspoon espresso powder, and milk into a bowl.
2. Whisk constantly for 2 minutes or until it is thick.
3. Take 4 paper cups or plastic drinking cups and divide the mixture equally into the paper cups.
4. Cover the cups with plastic wrap and place it in the refrigerator.
5. While the first layer is chilling, prepare the second layer.
6. Add condensed milk, vanilla extract, the rest of the espresso powder, and the cocoa powder into a bowl and whisk well. Add more espresso powder to taste if desired.
7. Add water and whisk until well combined.
8. Pour the condensed milk mixture over the chilled first layer.
9. Cover the paper cups with foil. Make a slit in each of the foil. Insert Popsicle sticks through the slit, into the cup.
10. Place the pudding pops in the freezer. Freeze until they are firm. It should take around 10 – 12 hours.
11. Just before serving, discard the foil and the paper cup as well.

AFTERWORD

By now you know more than enough to help you get started with the Sirtfood diet. You know how the sirtuin activators work. You know how it will benefit your body. Following the Sirtfood diet guidelines and using the recipes given in this guide will help you improve your overall health in no time.

Be sure to stay away from junk food and anything that you already know will push you back from your end goal. While it is okay to indulge in such foods occasionally, you need to avoid them as much as possible. Eating such foods too often will cut back on the benefits of the Sirtfood diet and only make you gain weight again. If you want to live a long and healthy life instead of one burdened with health issues, it is important to eat well, and even more so as you grow older.

Weight gain has many disadvantages that you may already have experienced like lack of energy, low self-confidence, high risk of diseases like diabetes type 2, etc. Switching over to a healthy Sirtfood diet and lifestyle plan will help you curtail such negative effects and lead a better life. It may be a little difficult at first, but the Sirtfood diet is a lot easier to

Afterword

follow than other fad diets. An added incentive to continue following it is that you will see real results.

There are many celebrities like Adele who have followed this diet and seen significant weight loss in recent years. If you are ready to experience such benefits for yourself, start implementing the guidelines of this diet in your own life now. If you find it effective, you can even recommend this book to other friends or family who could benefit from it.